For Endings to End Beginnings Have to Begin

By Teresa Moore

"One million people commit suicide every year"
World Health Organisation

Published by:
Chipmukapublishing
PO Box 6872
Brentwood
Essex
CM13 1ZT
United Kingdom

http://www.chipmunkapublishing.com

I thank everyone who I have met on my journey through life both good, bad and indifferent for they have helped shaped me into the person I am today.

Chapter I
The Early Years

My earliest memory is of my fourth birthday and my little sister opening my presents as little sisters do. Life at four was great. At weekends mum and dad took us to see nana and granddad and we'd have days at the zoo or go for picnics. I loved bonfire nights and dad would take us over the playing fields at the back of where we lived. Although mum didn't like fireworks we would wave to her as she looked out of the bedroom window whizzing our sparklers around and shouting with awe at the magnificent display of colour in the night sky.

There was always lots of laughter to be heard at home. I spent many hours during the summers playing with the caterpillars amongst the dandelion leaves and eating the sour apples from the next door neighbours tree then coming down with a bad case of the trots.

Christmas Eve would see a glass of sherry and a mince pie put out for Santa Clause and a carrot for Rudolph then bed. Christmas morning saw us running in to wake up mum and dad then dash down stairs to see if Santa had been. We always had a new coat off our nana and granddad who lived near the sea ready for the cold winter snow. Once all of the presents had been unwrapped we went round to nanas and granddads for dinner. The whole family was there and we'd all sit around the table for the feast of turkey followed by Christmas pud.

Every weekend mum took us to the phone box at the end of the road to speak to nana and granddad. My sister and I always argued over who was going to speak first. I remember my first day at school or rather going home crying because they hadn't taught me to read and write but it was okay because there was the next day and the next. At playtime the family dog would jump over the gate and come and see me (I didn't live far from the school) and then the teachers came and asked me to take him home, at which point mum usually ran up the road with his lead,   calling him.

May Day was always nice as mum went up into the meadow for the first of the may blossom for dad to decorate a maypole that I'd proudly march round the village with the rest of the children at my school. In the summer whilst dad was at work mum packed up a picnic and we ventured into the meadow not far from home. Then my sister and I played amongst the tall grasses with our dog and mum watched intently.

My aim was to become six years old. The school was a very small one so that everyone was in the same room and when you were six you got to sit at the back of the classroom and have a desk with a lid on it. This meant you could put your pencils, rubbers and reading books in it.   Sure enough I did become six and I did get to sit at the back of the classroom, mum and dad had even bought me new pencils and rubbers which I proudly placed in the desk on my first day. The next day however, my sister and I were told that we were moving house. I was really upset, as my time on the big desks which I had waited for so long had come to an abrupt end.

Chapter 2
Holidays

Our annual holiday was spent visiting our 'rich relatives' who lived near the sea. The journey was so long that most of it was spent sleeping, but as soon as we neared the coast dad woke us up for that first glimpse of the sea, which mum had smelled miles before. We sang with joy knowing that the next week would be full of treats and that we'd be spoilt rotten. Nan and granddad were always waiting at the front gate to greet us as we pulled up, to help us unload our suitcases from the car. Then once inside we'd catch up on the previous year's events. Nan and granddad always commented on how much my sister and I had grown over the last year. There was always plenty to eat and we'd play with our cousins in the garden where granddad grew marrows and grapes.

The week was crammed with day trips to the beach, making sandcastles and swimming in the sea with our cousins. Then on the way back to Nan and granddads we'd stop off for a tub of shellfish, which was devoured with great pleasure. One thing Nan always made sure of was that my sister and I had exactly the same as our cousins, who only lived in the next town to them. This meant that every time they had a chocolate bar over the year one was put away for us so that by the time it was holiday time again there would be bags and bags full of chocolate and sweets.

A lot of the time was spent with our cousins and aunts and uncles. I loved them dearly and always wished that they lived closer as I only saw them once a year. My uncle always teased us over our midlands accent saying that we didn't speak properly whilst our other uncle took pleasure in seeing who would scream first at his Chinese burns which he inflicted on our wrists. Then once we had screamed he would let go to reveal a huge red and sore mark where he had rubbed.

One day was always put aside during the holiday for the slot machines at the fair ground. I'd spend hours playing with the penny games and was always elated when the pennies dropped into the opening - never thinking of how many I'd put in to make them drop though! Night times were spent looking through photo albums of all the family as Nan always made sure she was updated regularly with snap shots of us all. Always a mug of milky-malted bournvita then I'd get tucked up in bed, as Nan would say "Night and bless."

Sometimes Granddad got us up out of bed really early and took us on the ranges where he worked after coming out of the army. This was called the 'rabbit run' because the whole point of it was to chase off the rabbits, which there were hundreds of. I always loved this but wished it didn't have to be done so early in the mornings.

At the end of the week the return journey was made back home and although I loved visiting my rich relatives and enjoyed the sea I was unceasingly elated to get home and back to normal.

Chapter 3
Confusion

The new house was bigger than the old one, which was good because it meant that there was more room to play. I loved my dolls and nana was always giving me materials to make new dresses. I'd started a new school a lot bigger than my old one but that was okay too as it gave me a chance to make new friends.

I remember when I was nine I desperately wanted to learn to play the flute. I had gone to see about having lessons at school but the peripatetic tutor said that I had the wrong shaped lips to play the flute, which I was really unhappy about. Dad went up to the school and asked if they could just give me a try, as I was so passionate about it – which they did.

Mum and dad took my sister and me to nanas and granddads every weekend without fail. Sometimes we'd play in the park. Granddad took us to the shop with ten pence each to buy sweets but we always came back with a lucky bag consisting of a toy, the pretend cigarettes and bubble gum. Then chomping on the gum dad complained that we had "bought that 'rommal' again!" and my sister and I sang "I Closed My Eyes", from Joseph and His Technicolor Dreamcoat to our family who clapped joyously at the rendition.

After demolishing a big dinner of roast beef and Yorkshire puds we walked along the 'cut' if the weather was nice and watched the men fishing. Nana kept an ear open for the first cuckoo of the year but I never heard it till later. Some weekends mum and dad let us stay at nanas and granddads overnight, which was a real adventure. That was until one morning when nana came in to get us up. She didn't sound her normal self and as

I looked up it became apparent why. She hadn't got any teeth in! I screamed the house down as I was so frightened, thinking Nan's teeth had fallen out over night but she reassured me that she had forgotten to put them in and that's she had false teeth for years and couldn't believe I had only just noticed.

Things started to feel different at home, I'd come in from playing or school and there was a tension in the air which was new to me. Mum and dad were always arguing and I hated the upheaval it was causing. I watched mum kick dad between the legs till he had to crawl up the stairs doubled up in agony and lie on the bed for a while. I couldn't cope with what happened at home and became behind with my schoolwork but because I didn't want my parents to know, I forged mum's signature on the homework book. Nobody suspected a thing - that was until I lost the book at school and it was sent home. I had been sprung but didn't feel able to say why I had done it, so I took the punishment given and promised it wouldn't happen again.

Then one-day and completely out of the blue, mum disappeared. Dad told us she had gone down to Nan and granddads for a holiday. For a while things returned to normal apart from mum not being there which I felt was down to me with the homework book.

Much of my time was taken up with my animals that I loved dearly. There were rabbits, guinea pigs and a dog that gave me rides. I'll never forget the day I went to feed my guinea pig and after opening the hutch running back into the house screaming as I thought there was a rat in there. It was discovered shortly after however, that it wasn't a rat but a baby guinea pig much to the whole family's joy.

The day mum returned from her holiday will always stick in my mind. She came to school and took me out of my history lesson because I was 'needed at home', I was dragged home and the door locked behind us. Nan and granddad were also there and suitcases had been packed and were on the doorstep. My sister wasn't allowed out of school early which in retrospect was a good thing. When dad came home from work he saw these suitcases on the doorstep. I was not allowed to let him in, nana's hand was put over my mouth and I was hidden so that dad couldn't see me. It was only when dad threatened to put a brick through the window to get in that I managed to wriggle free and shout out. I had no idea what was happening but I will never forget the look on his face when he saw me. I just wanted to let dad back into the house but I wasn't allowed to, I was angry and hurt as I watched my dad walk down the drive, suitcases in his hands and get in his car and drive off.

This was the beginning of a very traumatic two years. Dad wasn't home anymore so it was my mum, my sister and me.

Life was ok initially but before long it was clear that mum was weird! She'd say strange things and do bizarre stuff which I'd never seen before. On coming home from school I endeavoured to do the housework or start the tea. Mum was asleep on the sofa. Some nights mum woke me up because she was convinced someone had been murdered in the houses behind ours. On one occasion the police asked me questions in the small hours over something mum had come out with. I became very unhappy. We saw dad at weekends and wanted to be with him permanently because of what mum was saying and doing. So dad began a long battle to get custody of us.

After coming home from a friend's house one day, mum had a go at me because I had been writing on my hand. Although I tried to explain to her that it was a phone number she was adamant that it was a sign of the devil and we had to leave straight away as she felt we were no longer safe. She was also convinced that a friend of dads had placed drugs inside of us. So, in the middle of the night we packed our bags. Nan and granddad came and picked us up, animals as well, and I thought I would never see or speak to dad again.

Nan's house was near the sea so much of the time was spent on the beach. Back at the house I never understood what was happening as my relatives whispered amongst themselves. The atmosphere was very dense and I felt I was to blame even though I couldn't quite work out why and felt guilty that I had let my friend scribble her number on my hand. Although I had spent all my holidays at Nan's and her house felt like home, on this occasion it didn't and even though it was familiar I felt really uncomfortable, not having a clue what was happening. I was so upset that I wet the bed one night and was too afraid to tell anyone so I covered it up with the sheets and hoped no one would notice.

Mum spent much of her time arguing with the workmen doing maintenance work on the nearby road. She felt that they were interfering with her thought processes and she would be found. On another day we had gone into a café to eat, and just as the food was brought to the table a particular song came on the juke box, which mum said was a sign that she needed to go to Libya and marry Colonel Gaddafi. Abruptly, mum grabbed my sister and I just as we were about to tuck in to our much looked forward to egg and chips, and hurried us back to nana's house. It was utter chaos but after a week mum decided to take us home as she felt it was then safe to do so.

Life went from bad to worse. I lost my friends at school and became classed as the 'school gypo' who had a 'nutcase' for a mum.

People laughed at me walking down the street with mum because she talked to herself. I was bullied at school then would go home not knowing what I would walk into. I slept in my school clothes most of the time to reduce the washing load but in fact turned up for school smelly and unkempt. It was little wonder that I was picked on as much as I was. A sister who I had been very close to until now, began to blackmail me into doing things I really didn't want to do but mum stayed on the sofa asleep.

I was so relieved when the day came that dad won the custody battle and I didn't have to live with mum anymore. I hated mum so intensely and thought that now we were back with dad everything would be okay, and back to normal proper family again. All our clothes were packed up ready for the move. Dad had to get the house in order ready to be sold so he put everything else on a bonfire in the back garden. My toys, my first shoe and my christening gown all went up in flames along with many other possessions which could never be replaced.

Everything was gone.

Shortly after this we moved into our new house and dad got remarried. I thought this was great as I loved my stepmother dearly but things don't always go to plan!

Chapter 4
Family life

Following the trauma of the previous two years with mum I found it very difficult to settle back into family life as well as starting a new school. Dad wasn't the person I remembered which was really difficult. I yearned for him to hug me but it never happened so I learnt not to expect it. My sister was doing things which always resulted in my getting the blame, and I was beginning to find life hard going with my stepmother.

Although I put a lot of effort in to my schoolwork I was very unhappy and felt like school was my respite from my increasingly strained home life. After a while my unhappiness was picked up on at school and I was approached by one of my teachers. Unfortunately I couldn't really say much because I had been told that family problems were to stay within the family and not to go to 'outsiders'. I was advised to keep a diary as a way of getting my feelings out, which worked until it was found.

Arguments were a way of life at home and all too frequently I was the cause of them. If I answered back I was wrong, if quiet and blank I was wrong, and if I cried it was perceived that I was trying to emotionally blackmail my parents. Sometimes the arguments would last for hours and I felt so drained and felt the only way I could get through them was knowing that it would soon be time for school again.

After a while I began to harden off to the constant conflict with my parents albeit with difficulty especially because I found the concept of having to ask for everything very hard to accept. The biscuits were counted and if one was missing without being accounted for it was my fault every time. I never grasped asking to go to the toilet either, for when I did ask I was told I didn't have to, but when I forgot to ask another argument would unfold. Brick walls were beginning to be erected around me in order to survive the constant battles that I was faced with daily. And with every row, and every put down the wall became thicker and stronger and more difficult to penetrate.

Christmas was always strained and I never looked forward to holidays. The one statement dad always came out with was no matter what happened, 'you must always be yourself'. My problem was that when I was myself was when I got into the most trouble hence feeling constantly confused.

Most of the people my age at school were going to sleepovers and day trips which I felt unable to go to because that would mean having to ask permission from my parents. I found this particularly difficult as the past had taught me not even to bother asking in case an argument broke out, and I'd do anything to minimise the risk of provoking an argument.

At the age of fifteen I knew I was beginning to have real difficulty and asked to speak with a counsellor at school, but because of my age I was informed that this would not be possible without the involvement of my parents. I begged for this not to happen because I knew the outcome would be very grim. I did see a counsellor but only twice. The first time I tried to say how I felt but was so fearful of my parents finding out that I only mentioned the easier issues. Afterwards I was met with silence from my parents for quite a few days so when I went back the second time it was to tell him that things were okay and maybe there was nothing really wrong. I did this so that my parents would speak to me again.

I had come a long way with my flute and began to pass my grades swiftly resulting in my being competent enough to join the local wind band. I was in my element because music had become a way of life for me and I could never imagine living without it. I ate, drank and slept music and found this very beneficial as an outlet for many of my feelings that I found difficult to cope with at any given moment.

As time went on I became more and more introvert and spent the majority of my time in my own company, so that I couldn't say anything wrong to anybody and get comeback from it. I became emotionless, which was a survival measure but in the process lost sight of reality and what was happening around me. I'd also learnt that my mum was ill with schizophrenia which is why she had acted the way she had, and I had become angry with her. I had not seen her or heard from her in years and had hated her with such passion thinking that she was a horrible person when really it wasn't her fault. I began to regret the feelings of hate that I'd held close to my heart for many years when really she was not to blame. I felt awful, as I had no idea of where she was in the world and whether I'd ever see her again.

I ran away from home as I found it difficult to accept all these feelings that had come all together and I felt I needed time to myself to think. I walked and walked and for the first time ever I felt so free. The thought of no more arguments and conflicts was like a huge weight lifting from me and I didn't want it to end. I also knew however that a life on the streets was not in the equation, not for me at least, so I eventually dragged myself back home.

Life was particularly difficult as a result of my running away, especially on the family holiday. I had said sorry but my punishment meant that I was unable to cope because I had been banned from playing my flute. This in itself was soul destroying but combined with spending the majority of my time alone while my family went off sightseeing really hurt me. I spent my days sitting near the sea and wondering if there really was a chance of a life.

I desperately wanted a career in music but there were always barriers put in the way. My music teacher had made it clear that I needed a second instrument if I was going to make a career out of music, which I didn't have. Dad always said that I didn't need it, because one flute should be enough if I really wanted it. So, I bounced between my music teacher and dad until I had to make a decision, which eventually was made for me.

Chapter 5
Innocent Until Proven Guilty!

During my last year of 'A' levels my life took a turn which was far from expected. My life consisted of battles with my parents and much of the time fighting with my sister. I always felt she ended up getting the better deal even though it felt to me that I was the only person who saw beyond her façade. One day, shortly after my parents realised that my sister had not returned home from school, there was a knock on the door. It was the police, they had come to arrest both my dad and step mother on grounds of assaulting my sister and they were taken away for questioning. I sat at home wondering what was going on until their return very late that evening. When they explained that my sister had accused them of beating her up I was dumbfounded because although I had become very bitter towards them I knew that they would never lay a finger on either of us, especially my sister.

Literally hours after the first arrest the police came back to re-arrest dad who was subsequently charged with sexual assault. I couldn't understand why my sister said what she had. After this dad was re-arrested several times on different charges all surrounding abuse. As well as dad being arrested there were around twenty other families where someone was arrested, all supposedly involved in a paedophile ring. All of the children were taken into care while the investigation went on. The forensic officers came one day and it was like something out of a television programme, men in white body suits who took all the tapes and videos away in the hope that there would be some evidence.

Although this was directly aimed at dad, I found it particularly difficult as I still attended the same school as my sister. I always tried my hardest to avoid engaging in conversation but my sister constantly spitting in my face made this more difficult and I felt powerless. Even more so when my nana phoned me up asking me to back up my sister but because I knew it was untrue I told her I couldn't, to which she replied 'You're no granddaughter of mine' and hung up.

Also during this time dad had a phone call from social services asking if they thought his ex-wife, my mum, was capable of looking after a baby as she had a son who was a few days old. I screamed down the phone and begged dad to say no. He felt unable to do this and answered that she could, but only with 24 hour supervision and thus a new contact was made between mum and me and now my half brother.

I had made a decision about my career and felt that it was time for me to do something with my music, and the Royal Air Force felt like the answer I was searching for, so I applied to become a bands woman. I took all of the aptitude tests required which I found really easy and went down to an Air Force base for my practical audition. I was absolutely devastated when they said that I was just a little too young and to re-apply in a year where they would reconsider me.

Chapter 6
The Mental Health System and Me

I entered the mental health system when I was 18 years old, during the period of allegations involving my sister and my dad. After spending a night on the streets, and by mutual agreement with my GP, I was admitted to the local psychiatric hospital for a 'rest'. Before I had chance to breathe however I was informed that I was depressed and was prescribed Prozac. I don't remember much about my early years in the system, other than my admissions to hospital being very traumatic. I was always trying different cocktails of medications and spent much of my time on the ward trying to run away, usually because I felt frightened and not listened to.

My first experience of a psychiatric hospital was filled with terror as the building itself dated back to the years of the old lunatic asylum. I had heard many stories from my Nanna about when she was a little girl and how her parents made her stay inside when the sirens went off and the men in white coats came knocking on the doors to warn of an escapee, and to be on guard and not to approach these people because they were said to be violent and dangerous. In reality, and when I was admitted, I was pleasantly surprised to discover that these were just ordinary people living their life only experiencing problems and needing help to get better.

Once settled in and an inventory completed I spent the majority of the time there within the grounds and mingling with the other patients, it was a community in itself. The main building consisted of a maze of corridors and it was easy to get lost. There was a canteen where all the patients from the different wards met at mealtimes. The hospital was self sufficient in every way even having a hairdresser and dentist, and surrounding the main building were many smaller buildings including a locked ward. I found my first ward review very daunting, going in with the expectation of there being only a psychiatrist and a bed to lie on to talk about your problems. In reality I was shocked when I walked into a room to find it cram packed with faces that I had never seen before. It was so overwhelming, especially as no one had prepared me for what was behind the ward review door.

My thoughts were of really wanting some help in order to get my life back on track so that I could continue with my exams, yet in the review I felt my needs were not the focus for discussion. All the people in this tiny room were far more interested in seeing if they could trip me up into admitting the allegations my sister had come up with were true. I left the review feeling extremely angry at being ignored and not heard, and yet again the focus being concentrated on my sister who wasn't even there!

During a later admission to the hospital the psychiatrist decided that due to the symptoms I was exhibiting he reached a diagnosis of schizophrenia and I was put on depot injections. I didn't really notice any difference in myself on the depots other than I didn't think much, If I did have a moment where I thought and found it really difficult my meds were altered. I didn't think I was schizophrenic but thought that it might mean I would be given help, as I knew something wasn't right.

At one stage of another admission I ran away from the ward and was sectioned, which meant that I had to stay there for three days and they put me on the secure ward, which was awful. I couldn't even go to the toilet without asking and it felt like a prison. There were a lot of very ill people there and I felt like I didn't fit in and couldn't understand why they had put me there for running away. Whereas the other people there were drugged up I wasn't, which made it even harder.

On admission to this ward I had asked if they could inform my parents but found out that this was not done until the second day.

I also began to experience some side effects due to the depots I was on but it took two hours of persuading the staff that I hadn't received my tablets before they went to find my card to see that indeed, it hadn't been administered. I think the hardest part was knowing that they didn't believe a word I said because I was a 'mental patient' and then, to rub salt into the wound, I was asked if I wanted to watch a video which I thought was a good idea in order for the day to go a bit quicker. It was much to the nurses' amusement when they saw my face as the great escape music came on the television and I was subjected to the whole of this film from beginning to end.

My life was taken up with depot clinics; drop in centres and hospital and before long I was in the system in a big way. If I felt unhappy my meds could be increased until I felt that I couldn't survive without them. When things got too much for me I would be admitted to hospital where I had chance to get stabilised.

Hospital felt safe. Apart from not having the responsibility of cooking and cleaning there were people around constantly if you wanted to talk. I found this a novelty and to a degree comforting. There was never a dull moment on the ward and if I couldn't cope I was allowed extra tablets to block out the feelings. I became a regular at the hospital along with many others and started to build up a network of friends. Our conversations consisted of meds and their side effects, and what the nurses were getting wrong.

When I was twenty two I got married to a man who I had met through my admissions to hospital. Here was someone who accepted me and unconditionally loved me and although I thought the world of him it only lasted a year.

During this year I ended up getting sterilised without any form of pre-op counselling because of the pressure put on me by my husband and my family, yet at the time I had no concept of the enormity of this as I really thought that I would be ill forever, so in some ways it would serve me practically. I felt like I was being held back and I wanted the opportunity to work and see life other than the four walls of the flat, but we were worlds apart and so I walked out on him.

Due to being homeless I ended up in a women's refuge. The staff there was aware of my diagnosis and I did feel as if I was patronised as a result. Confirmation of this came when I asked to use the computer to type up an official letter. Before I did it I had asked the staff to read it to make sure it contained the relevant information. I had surprised them by my articulate and succinct manner within the contents of the letter because they hadn't realised that I was capable of having a brain, as well as being mentally ill. I found this particularly difficult to comprehend, as I was in no doubt of my intellectual capacity and frustrated that I had been judged on a diagnosis rather than me as a person.

I found myself a new boyfriend who was nearly thirty years older than me but I didn't feel that the age gap was a problem and I loved him dearly. We spent our time travelling around from place to place and he'd buy me gift upon gift. I loved the attention which I was getting and thought that we were going to be together forever.

During our relationship I started going to church where I found an inner peace which I hadn't felt before, and began to get involved more by going regularly and also attending study groups. My boyfriend found this particularly difficult to handle because I had found something I enjoyed doing other than being with him. He started to walk me to and from church and if I was a minute later than I'd said he would begin to argue with me. I was no longer allowed to cook or clean or do anything that gave me a sense of who I was and I began to dread coming out of church as I never knew what sort of reception I would get.

Things began to go seriously wrong when my boyfriend started to dope me up with diazepam so that he could sleep with me, sometimes having to carry me up the stairs as I was so doped up. He knew I'd put up a fight so as I became immune to the tablets he would increase the dose. If I resisted life was made even worse than it already was. I hadn't got the right communication skills to let people know what was happening so I arranged to walk away from the relationship and away from the area so I couldn't be found

Chapter 7

Life with Borderline Personality Disorder

As time went on my behaviour became more and more bizarre, and the medication began to have little effect. The relationship became more difficult to cope with and it didn't help matters when I found myself being abused in a voluntary job I had taken on. I spent my time ringing round help lines but I found them unhelpful or unapproachable until I spoke to someone on the rape crisis helpline and for the first time ever I felt like I was being heard. It was little comfort being on the end of a phone as I still had to live through what was happening more and more frequently. The counsellor began sending me cards and taking a real interest in me and I was beginning to realise that I was not schizophrenic, after years of being convinced and then convincing myself.

After leaving the abusive relationship I ended up in a hospital out of my local area, which meant new nurses who had never met me before and had no pre- conceived ideas of who I was. The psychiatrist observed me for a while and decided that I did not have schizophrenia, but had Borderline Personality Disorder. I remember going back to my regular clinic so pleased that I hadn't got a mental illness but was told that it was a worse diagnosis than schizophrenia - because it couldn't be treated. On top of this I had made the realisation that I was gay and although at the time I felt this to be quite a revelation I had a lot to learn!

Nothing could have prepared me for what was to lie ahead. Although I had no
concept of the enormity of such a label I knew that it wasn't a mental illness and thus didn't need psychotropic meds so after seven years, I came off them.

I felt that I was ignored, not listened to. The professionals took a different view of me now I had a new label. The word 'untreatable' bounced around my head, and I did become a difficult case. My life now existed from crisis to crisis, I began to self-harm to the point where I was playing 'Russian Roulette' and I would be admitted to A&E or the psychiatric hospital on a daily basis. I was taking different cocktails of prescribed medication, and the doses were becoming ever greater.

People were treating me like a leper which I didn't understand. On one occasion I had overdosed and been admitted to A&E but because I was a regular I was treated with contempt to the point that when they discharged me I had no shoes on and no money. Home was two buses away, which I made them aware of and I still had to leave. It was really humiliating walking into the nearby town bare foot not knowing how I was to get home. The police picked me up and gave me a lift home much to a lot of people's warped sense of humour.

On another occasion I had been admitted to hospital because I couldn't cope with the fact that my step-dad had died. While sitting in the lounge one day a man came in. It was the man who had abused me badly so I went down to my room to pack my stuff up. There was no way I could stay in a place where he was allowed to sleep under the same roof, so I told the staff what I was doing and they agreed to transfer him to another unit. I stayed in my room until I was told that he had gone and was persuaded to go back up to the day area, but when I did finally go up they had lied to me for he was sitting in the smoke room as if nothing had happened. I became so angry that they thought that I wouldn't notice him that I discharged myself.

I became really distressed and my self harm had reached a peak because I felt it was the only way people could see I was hurting as I had given up on words years ago. I began to become more and more determined that I didn't want to live like this and thought my only option was death as I was 'untreatable' and 'a difficult case,' which I soon became.

I remember overdosing and then seeing the GP within literally hours of being discharged from hospital. I told him what I'd done so he prescribed me another three months supply of the same drug. I was so angry that I had not been heard that I took the lot and ended up going into spasm. I came round a few days later in hospital yet again.

People became increasingly hostile towards me so I became more hostile towards the world. I was angry, confused and scared. I was out of control and felt very alone. The hospital where I had once found safety became cold and threatening. I wanted help desperately, but no one was listening. I didn't like who I had become but knew no way out until I heard about a Therapeutic Community and I knew it was the only answer so I sought referral.

Whilst waiting for the referral to be processed I reached rock bottom. I decided that the only answer was to kill myself so I went to throw myself out of my flat on the top floor. The police bashed my door down and took me to be assessed but I was deemed to be of sound mind and I was allowed to go home. Unfortunately, during the process I lost my cross and became very upset. I went down to the station next day to say that I had found my cross, with a view to hiding somewhere and killing myself. The police officer saw that I had a knife and came towards me; I became frightened and ended up threatening him as he got too close to me which resulted in my being taken to the cells.

All the feelings came flooding back of the police involvement from years before and thinking that this was how dad was treated only he was innocent. I was guilty. I had to strip down to my pants and wear a bodysuit which was awful especially as I was on my period at the time. This meant that every time I needed to freshen up I had to ask for my toiletries and was watched whilst I did it. I couldn't stop crying as I just wanted a cigarette which I was eventually allowed but felt it unfair when the other people in the custody cells were allowed one every time they asked for one. They were swearing all the while but I felt that gave them respect but I couldn't do that as I felt so ashamed at what had happened, but as a result got treated really badly in comparison.

It was decided that I wasn't fit for interviewing that night so I had to wait until the following morning. I asked for a drink but it never came and at one point I thought an officer was coming towards me ready to give me a punch until someone else went past and he retracted his hand.

I was charged with possessing an offensive weapon and threats to kill, which I could not deny, as it was the truth. My time in the cell was horrific in the extreme and when I was released on bail it was to the local psychiatric hospital and I vowed things had got to change. I was there for the first week of my bail and after a day the realisation of what had happened really struck home. I sat outside the unit and began to cry. The tears were never ending as my emotions got all muddled up and confused. I don't remember ever crying as intensely as this before. One of the nurses came out to see if I was alright, to which I replied that I was okay and just needed to cry, and I wasn't in any danger of self harming as I just hadn't got it in me. When I went back to my room I found that it had been stripped of all my belongings so I went marching up to the staff room, I was so angry! It was bad enough that I'd been stripped of my dignity at the police station without the same happening here, as I felt it was so unnecessary. After a week I returned home. It was awful because I had letters upon letters from my neighbours asking me to kill myself, as they didn't want me living around them and their children any longer. I found this difficult to understand as I never did anything in front of people though the cuts on my arms were enough to frighten them.

Whilst waiting for the case to come to court I was re-arrested for an alleged attack which I had not done, on someone I had confided in about my case, and I found it really difficult to prove I hadn't done it but I was not charged.

The therapeutic community which I had already been referred to seemed further away than ever as I thought I had blown my chances. But as I received a conditional discharge I was still eligible for it so I went through the selection process and managed to get a place. All I remember saying on selection was that I wanted to live instead of exist but not really having any concept of what was to happen. I felt that this was my last chance.

Chapter 8
My Last Chance

I didn't know or like myself so I was damned if anybody else was going to but I desperately wanted the hurting, emptiness and anger to stop but I didn't know how to do it and I hated the world.

When I was accepted into the Therapeutic Community I didn't have time to think just how much it would change my life, it was such a culture shock. Nothing could have prepared me for the roller coaster of emotions I was about to experience. I was determined to complete the therapy, which was one year residential, although it was difficult to stay most of the time.

Whilst there I saw 'acting out' in different forms and realised how I looked to the world. I slowly learned just what an impact my behaviour had on people over the years, to which I had been totally oblivious before. There were reasons why I had behaved in that way at the time, but I began to realise that these were inappropriate responses.

I began to learn to understand my emotions and why I felt like I did, in a supportive environment (although it didn't always feel supportive) I learned to trust people. Even with the fear of rejection always present I was able to discard all my masks to find out who I really was.

I learned to cry, and there were lots of tears, I learned to genuinely care for others without thinking what was in it for me. I learned to laugh, which was an amazing experience. I learned to verbalise my anger rather than smashing myself up or becoming verbally aggressive. I learned that crying was a normal response to situations but most of all I was listened to and I learned to like myself, which gave me enough self-respect, and also develop awareness for those around me. I learned that the way you behave can affect other people's attitudes towards you.

I was listened to and I began to find a voice which I had never thought possible, to the point where I fought to leave the Therapeutic Community two months early. It wasn't easy. It was slowly becoming acceptable to show my emotions and after years of having them covered up with medications I was starting to understand them. Things became less extreme in my life, and the daily crises became less and less as I began to live in the 'grey' - the middle ground - rather than the black and white I was used to.

The last 2 weeks of therapy were actually the hardest 2 weeks of my life as I began to realise what the therapy had been about. I always thought it was to deal with and come to accept your problems, but I realised there was one thing I had never faced before and that was saying 'Goodbye'. Goodbye to people you have been to hell and back with. Goodbye to the past - past experiences and past behaviours. And the months prior to that had prepared me to do something I had never done before. To grieve for all the years I had lost, but knowing I no longer needed to live in the past, I have a present and a future.

Chapter 9
Bah Humbug!

When I found myself back in the outside world it was as if I had woken up after a long sleep and found myself in a different country having to speak a new language. The practical is always different from the theory, which I learned fast but I was determined to speak this new language and be heard. In the early days it was really hard, as people would go on what I had been, instead of who I was now. I'd ended up in the same hostel I'd started in when I first left home. It had not changed in many ways and I felt like it was a re-run of previous but this was the chance I needed to get my life right and on track. I joined a new church, which I had a good feeling about so all was well.

My first Christmas that I had found 'me' was distinctly difficult. I'd hoped that my dad would ask me to spend it with him as I had hoped every year since I left home. Like every other year this didn't happen and as Christmas approached I spent my time growing more and more resentful of him. I thought that now that I had changed that it would naturally follow suit that my family would change. Obviously this was not the case. I yearned desperately to have my family back but soon realised that I could change me but not those around me. I was heart broken to discover that if dad wanted to change it would be up to him for no matter how different I was it was achieved because I wanted it. Dad, it seemed, was happy with the way he was and saw no need to change. It felt like he didn't realise he still had a daughter. It was a hard lesson to learn and I shed many tears in the process.

I went to my new church for some of the Christmas services until the day I felt I could not return. This was when I had decided to leave during the service and ended up being followed by people who I didn't even know. They would not let me leave the building as I was told that I had the devil in me and it needed getting rid of. Then they restrained me as I tried to leave and exorcise me. I felt like I was being spiritually raped. It was awful. All of these people holding on to me and saying things that were so far from the truth it was unreal. If I spoke up their voices just increased in volume so I just let them do what they felt they had to do and then when it was all over I left feeling very raw and hurting deeply. How could I trust any Christian again?

Chapter 10
Prince's Trust Personal Development Programme

My time on the Prince's Trust Volunteers Personal Development Programme was far from easy.

From the day I joined I had to overcome a lot of personal barriers and this was a struggle at times. I did put a lot of pressure on myself due to the fact that that I had been given this opportunity and I wanted to make the most of it knowing it was my perhaps my last chance to do something like this. Being older than the rest of the team bought its own difficulties as I had to learn how to manage a flat as well as complete the programme, which at time meant long hours and lots of travelling as well as learning to weigh up priorities in order to achieve a future, as well as keep my flat going.

I felt so much older than the team to begin with, which included being wiser in a lot of ways. In the early days I was so envious of the interpersonal skills a lot of the team had and I knew I lacked because I had never really experienced anything other than institutions. P.T.V was a new world to me but one which I wanted to be part of so desperately that I embraced the whole programme with both arms and promised myself that whatever happened I would see it through to the end. Every day brought a new and different challenge either for me as an individual or the way in which I had to learn to interact with other people.

Residential proved very difficult and a very testing time but by the time I was climbing the rock face I began to realise that this was the start of something I had never before experienced in any great depth – life.

I was given opportunities which had never before been open to me, or perhaps I wasn't open to them, but my confidence was growing all the time.

I had no idea that I had leadership skills but I was actively encouraged to develop these with the full support of team leader. As the programme went on and the work involved was getting more intense I began to grow stronger and believe in myself so that although the course was tough I began to find it easier as I learnt not to beat myself up over minor problems.

By the time my individual placement was through my thinking had changed considerably and was more able to hear other people but not take it all on myself and thus overloading.

There was a real sense of low spirits in the team before the challenge, and I do remember a remark made to me about being the stronger one out of the volunteers at that time, which was a surprise to me as my thoughts had began to reach turmoil point as I knew the end was looming. I was under a considerable amount of pressure in those final weeks but I held myself together and carried things through to the very end.

I put every reserve into the course and pushed myself to the limits and beyond at times to see just what I was really capable of but I couldn't have done it without the support of the team leader. This was important to me, feeling safe enough to push myself all the way and if I did take a step back which happened in the earlier days I knew that I had someone along side me who would help me get back to my feet. Just knowing that at times was enough for me not to always end up falling and what helped me stand tall and eventually walk forward with my head held high.

On completing the Prince's trust programme I then went on to do two hundred hours as a millennium volunteer. I did this at the drop in centre where I'd done my placement on the team. It really opened my eyes being a professional in the same system that I had just left and I began to take a slightly different slant on life and indeed the system. I realised that the professionals, one of whom I had become, were human with their own problems and baggage. I had never seen this before! I also began to understand why rules were put in place. I got a real buzz from being part of the system but in a different capacity as I attended staff meetings, organised events and under went supervisions.

I loved being around the members and became extremely passionate about defending people with mental health issues. After all I'd been one of them myself. Whereas most of the staff could only sympathise I was able to empathise which made for a good working relationship with both my colleagues and the members, and at times put a slightly different slant on discussion.

As far as I was concerned I was no longer a service user in the system but a professional. Had I come a long way!

My time apart from work was taken up with attending award ceremonies resulting in my gaining the volunteer achievement award both locally and regionally. I was in my element when I accepted these awards standing so proudly giving a speech as to how I had come to get them. I felt in some way that I was sticking my fingers up to the system which had said that I was untreatable and I did this with such confidence.

I'd made it. All the fighting to stay afloat had paid off as I enjoyed my newly found self. I knew that what ever was presented to me through the rest of my life would be dealt with and I would never have to go back to the system as a user as I had conquered my personality disorder and that was that!

Chapter 11
Not in my control!

Once my millennium hours had been completed I continued at the centre until I started college. I had decided to get my teaching certificate and I chose to facilitate mental health awareness workshops in order to gain this qualification. I found the course itself very interesting as much of the time was focused on the psychology behind teaching. When I began to do the workshops I realised that I had found my niche.

Unfortunately when I first started college I came down with a chest infection. I was determined not to let it affect my performance in the classroom so I ignored it for as long as I could. Even when I spent half the night in the local hospital being nebulised I would attend college the next day and carry on regardless. Dosed up with steroids and antibiotics I continued to deliver the workshops.

Suddenly my perception on life began to alter which again I tried to ignore. My whole world turned upside down as I began to feel people really touching me but no one was there, and everyone really was out to get me and trap me, and it became increasingly difficult to continue at college as my concentration went out the window.

I began to hear voices, which were unlike anything I had ever experienced before and my sense of reality seemed to be slipping away from me with every second to the point where I ended up being admitted to hospital. I couldn't believe what was happening and found it impossible to comprehend ending up in a place, which no longer felt safe and where I felt that I no longer belonged.

It was said that I was having a bad reaction to the steroids, which gave me a little comfort in knowing that it wouldn't be a permanent state. I could only rationalise what was happening by comparing what was going on to my time in the therapeutic community. Knowing that the structure would be of no help to me as the things that were happening were really not of my own doing. This frightened me as it was unknown territory and I didn't know how to deal with it.

After a few days I couldn't cope any longer with being in hospital. I discharged myself but agreed to have some support from a community psychiatric nurse. I was ambivalent though especially after my previous experiences with them.

Chapter 12
Merry Christmas!

At the age of twenty-eight I spent Christmas with my mother and brother for the first time since I was ten. I really looked forward to it as I really needed a break and thought it the perfect opportunity to do so as well as catch up with mum. I hoped the sea air would help my chest finish recovering and the thought of being with family for Christmas was amazing. I hadn't seen mum or my brother in nearly five years so there was a lot of catching up to do. From the moment I arrived I wanted to make the most of my time. It was difficult communicating with my brother as my French was limited and so was his English but mum acted as translator. It felt even stranger being caught up in sibling rivalry at my age on my brother's part but kind of nice.

I realised what I had craved over many years was to feel part of a family and here I did and yet another little bit of the jigsaw was fitted. My brother and mum only had one present each under the tree and they were from me. I began to realise how unimportant material possessions were and the emotional ties I had longed for for so long were fulfilled from the instant I got off the plane. I saw much of me in my brother from when I was his age right up to the present day and felt sad when mum told me she thought he needed medication to control his angry outbursts. I made it clear that it wasn't tablets he needed but firm boundaries to know where he stood as well as knowing he was loved and cared for which mum did take on board.

When I left was a really sad day and as I boarded the plane I had to choke back the tears not just of the week but of finding yet another part of me, the real me.

Chapter 13
Never say Never.

On my return from mum's I had a lot of emotion to deal with which wasn't easy, as a lot of it was new to me. My chest deteriorated and yet again I found myself being nebulised but the hardest thing to swallow was the psychosis setting in with vengeance. I tried to ignore it but it was clear it wasn't going to go away until finally I had to admit what was happening. Among the paranoia and delusions there was a part of me that recognised that I could lose my life if things carried on the way they were and after fighting so hard to find me I was really scared of losing it back to a hostile system which I knew too well.

This time I was heard by the professionals and had their full support in helping me to stay away from hospital which wasn't easy as I was convinced that they were conspiring to get me back in the system out of malice. I soon realised that you must never say never.

I went into hospital which I really did not want to do because of the experiences I'd had in the past. I was devastated – I felt that I had failed as a person and that although the BPD was not evident and I was indeed suffering a mental illness it was a bitter pill to swallow. What I couldn't see was that the system was rooting for me to get well and back on my feet to continue my journey that I had already started.

Where ever I go in life I will always have a piece of paper on file with the BPD label on which society looks on me as 'untreatable' but I KNOW DIFFERENT and I hope that this will be recognised with time.

When I look back on my life – living from crisis to crisis - just existing, it saddens me. There were times when I felt really let down by the mental health system and believed that if I had been listened to things may have been different but we can't live on 'what ifs'. The most horrific experience of my life, getting in trouble with the police, for which I still feel very ashamed, has turned out to be the turning point needed for me to take control of my life.

I have gone from being an 'untreatable' and 'difficult case' who played Russian roulette, who was angry and hurt and unhappy and who lived from admission to admission, instead I am now a balanced individual who has been nominated for three awards and is leaving the mental health system as a patient to rejoin it as a professional.

No matter where I go through life there are 10 years of files regarding my mental health and stating my untreatibility, but I am more than a diagnosis and truly believe that actions do speak louder than words. I was a victim who became a survivor but now I've conquered and continue to do so on a daily basis. There is life beyond 'Borderline Personality Disorder' and I'm witness to that!

Equally, I have learnt to never say never for there isn't one of us alive that can't experience mental ill health and it can strike at any time.

I really thought that as I'd conquered my BPD, I was immune to mental ill health but that wasn't so. So now I live from second to second and deal with whatever life throws at me as it happens but the one saying that will always remain with me and is so true is that **for endings to end beginnings have to begin.**